Gout Hater's Cookbook II

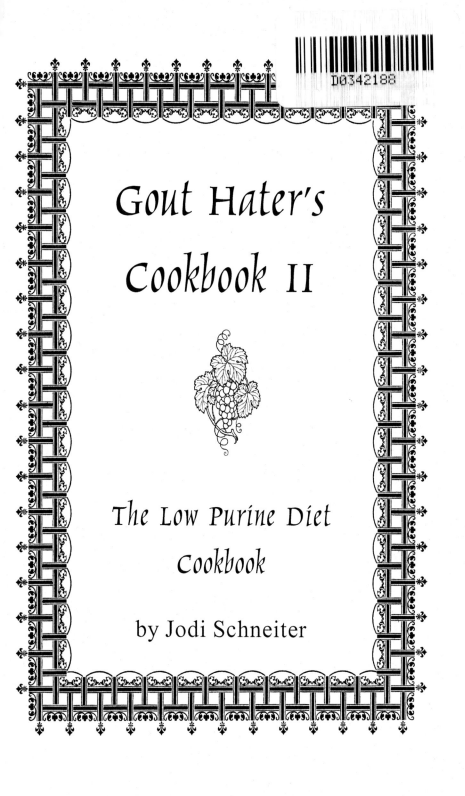

The Low Purine Diet Cookbook

by Jodi Schneiter

Gout Hater's Cookbook II
The Low Purine Diet Cookbook

Published by:
Reachment Publications
79 Whittington Drive
Palm Coast, Florida 32164
USA
Phone (386) 447-0324
Fax (386) 446-7579
Website: www.gout-haters.com

Library of Congress Control Number: 2001119328

ISBN: 1-888141-80-8

Please note: The contents of this book are in no way intended for use as a substitute for medical advice. Always consult your physician before making any changes in your diet. The information provided may vary from the regimen given to you by your physician or dietitian. As every individual case is different, please follow your recommended regimen, including diet and medications.

Many thanks to the Purine Research Society
and its efforts to help children with purine autism.

Special thanks to Dr. Robert C. Bennett
for his creative gourmet contributions.

Table of Contents

Introduction

Gout Hater's Cookbook II:
The Low Purine Diet Cookbook

Finding foods and recipes that will work with your prescribed diet can be difficult, especially when you have been placed on a regimen lower in purines.

Vegetarian burgers, for example, should be something anyone can eat. Unfortunately, most vegetarian burgers contain soy beans, which are legumes, and therefore not allowed on the restricted purine diet.

Spinach is another prime example. Although this leafy vegetable is rich in iron, riboflavin (vitamin B-2) and vitamin A, it is not allowed on the restricted purine diet.

However, limiting your diet to a given set of foods can open the door to a great number of healthy, delicious possibilities.

Once you begin to set aside the idea that you are being kept from the things you love, and begin concentrating on new recipes and flavors using ingredients you can safely eat, you will discover an infinite realm of wonderful foods.

Gout Hater's Cookbook II is second in the series of books designed to help you begin your adventure in restricted purine cuisine.

Our first book, *Gout Hater's Cookbook, Recipes Lower in Purines and Lower in Fat*, is based on the *modified* purine diet, which allows a moderately small amount of meat and some foods relatively high in purines.

Book II concentrates more on the *restricted* purine diet, which has been used by gout patients as well as families of children with purine autism. Dishes are based on the provided food lists, featuring a delicious ovo-lacto- (eggs and milk allowed) vegetarian diet. These recipes comply with both the modified and restricted purine diets. Fat and cholesterol are also avoided in efforts to accommodate persons with additional health issues.

The recipes in *Book II* were constructed in an effort to demonstrate just how wonderfully you and your family can eat, even on a restricted purine diet, while continually helping to lower your uric acid levels.

Your tastebuds, your doctor and your body will thank you.

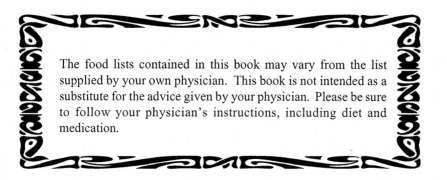

The food lists contained in this book may vary from the list supplied by your own physician. This book is not intended as a substitute for the advice given by your physician. Please be sure to follow your physician's instructions, including diet and medication.

Foods Allowed
(Lowest in Purines)

Beets (except beet tops), broccoli, carrots, celery, corn, cucumbers, eggplant, green string beans (not bulging), grits, hominy, jicama, leafy greens (except those not allowed), leeks, lettuce, okra, olives, onions, parsnips, peppers, potatoes, radishes, rhubarb, sago, squash, tomatoes, turnips, vegetable soups,[1] water chestnuts

Fruits, berries and fruit juice (except those not allowed)

Nuts (except peanuts - see Legumes, page 6)

Dairy (low fat or fat free): cottage cheese, cheese, eggs (no more than one yolk per day; more than one white is allowed), ice cream, margarine, milk, ricotta, yogurt. Watch the ingredients for xanthan/xanthum gum or xanthine.

Cereals (except whole grain); corn flakes

Semolina pasta/macaroni (preferably 100% semolina), white rice, tapioca

White flour (without malted barley flour added), matzoh, white rice flour, arrowroot flour, baker's yeast [2]

Ketchup, mustard, mayonnaise, honey, sugar

White bread, French bread, matzoh, plain white bagels (watch for malt), white pita bread

Sodas, non-cola, non-caffeine

Vegetable oils:[3] Canola, olive, soy

---

1. Not containing meat stock, meat extracts or high-purine vegetables.
2. Only as a part of baking. Yeast supplements are not allowed.
3. Peanut oil is not allowed.

FOODS AND INGREDIENTS
NOT ALLOWED

Foods Relatively High in Purines
Although excluded in this book's recipes, it is possible your system will be able to tolerate about 3 ounces of the following foods up to two times per week (check with your physician or dietician):

Artichokes, Asparagus, beans[1], bean sprouts, beet tops, bok choy, Brussels sprouts, cabbage, cauliflower, dried beans and peas, kale, legumes (page 6), lentils, mushrooms, peanuts and peanut butter, peanut oil, peas, soy/soy products (including tofu, soy sauce and soy flour)[2] spinach, Swiss chard

Wheat germ and whole grain cereal or flour, including barley, barley malt, bran, brown rice, oatmeal, oats, rye, pumpernickel, graham flour, malt, whole wheat, whole wheat flour; macaroni products not labeled as semolina or semolina durum

Meat, including beef, beef brisket, beef filet, beef chuck, cod, corned beef, crayfish, eel, haddock, lobster, mackerel, oyster, plaice, pike, pork, rabbit, shrimp, skinless white meat chicken or turkey, sole, meat broth, veal

Foods Highest in Purines
The following foods and ingredients are either very high in purines or otherwise not allowed in the restricted purine diet (Additional Notes, page 8):

Alcohol

Anchovies, caviar, fish roe, herring, mackerel, mussels, ocean perch, sardines, scallops, smelt, sprat, trout

Brains, game meats, horse, kidney, lamb, meat extracts/stock, organ meats, sausage, soups made from meat stock or extracts, spleen, tongue

Avocados, bananas, coconuts, seeds

Coffee, tea, chocolate, cocoa, cola drinks, carob, carob bean gum, caffeine

Brewer's yeast, yeast supplements, MSG, xanthine/xanthan gum, B-6 supplements, lard, powdered or evaporated milk, whole milk/milk products

---

1.Green string beans are allowed.
2. Soy oil is allowed.

Additional Notes

Soy products (not allowed) include tofu, soy flour and soy sauce. Soy oil is OK.

Whole grain cereal and flour includes barley, barley malt, bran, brown rice, pumpernickel, oatmeal, oats, rye, whole wheat, and macaroni products not labeled as semolina or semolina durum. Flour and pasta should be 100% semolina, which is more refined. Durum semolina is OK. 100% Durum is not OK.

Watch for xanthine, xanthan gum and unspecified vegetable gums when choosing cottage cheese, ice cream, ricotta and yogurt.

Watermelon and mangos should be limited to no more than one 1-inch slice per day.

Salicylates (such as aspirin) are not allowed (see page 103).

Green string beans are an immature bean and therefore allowed in this diet. However, only use them while the beans are very small and not bulging.

Avoid malt when choosing breads and cereals.

Eggs should be limited to one yolk per day. More than one egg white is OK.

Cheese should be limited to two ounces per day, one ounce each at separate times during the day.

Avoid extreme changes in diet. Fasting or severe dieting can raise your uric acid level and worsen or trigger an attack of gout. Dehydration can also provoke an attack. Be sure to drink lots of water.

When using vanilla extract, be sure to use only when the alcohol will be cooked out. Remember: virtually all extracts contain alcohol and should not be used in recipes that do not involve cooking out the alcohol content.

Alcohol and Nicotine

Avoid alcohol!!! Not only can alcohol contribute to an attack of gout, it is also possible that the affects of allopurinol are inhibited by alcohol intake.

If you are a smoker, try to reduce your nicotine intake. Nicotine is an extremely toxic substance which affects the central nervous system and causes an increase in heartbeat and breathing rates.

When used in conjunction with alcohol, the amount of addiction is said to increase. Among the immediate related effects, there is increased blood pressure. Long term effects include high blood pressure, which can ultimately cause gout.

Questions and Answers

What is gout?

Gout is brought on by the body's inability to eliminate excess uric acid, a by-product of purines.

This excess uric acid builds up in the form of needle-like crystals, usually around joint spaces or connective tissue. The build-up causes inflammation, redness, swelling and excruciating pain, so intense that even the touch of a bed sheet can be torture.

Attacks can occur overnight, and can be brought on by a shock or stress to the system, such as dehydration or alcohol consumption.

More than 2.1 million people in the United States suffer from gout. Gout can be acquired or inherited. Most cases (about 90%) occur in men over 40. Cases in women are usually seen after menopause.

Causes of hyperuricemia (excess uric acid in the blood) can be related to: hypertension, diuretic medication, use of low dose aspirin, renal insufficiency, obesity, extreme changes in diet, trauma, dehydration, alcohol consum-ption, surgery, and a diet of foods high in purines.

Treatments include preventive and symptom-relieving medicines, limited alcohol consum-ption and a diet of low-purine foods. Indeed, gout is said to be the only rheumatic disease known to be helped when certain foods are avoided.

What are purines?

Purines are a class of chemical compounds, with various derivatives containing a variation of the same basic structure. Included in this group are guanine and adenine, which are components of nucleic acids.

All naturally occurring purines are a variation on the same basic structure. Derivatives or structurally related compounds include theophylline and caffeine.

Purines play a variety of important roles in the system: For example, they act as messengers in cellular signaling for muscle contraction and nerve conduction. They help rid cells of excess nitrogen.

Purines act as antioxidants, helping to protect cells from agents which cause cancer. In addition, they work as the information molecules in genes, helping to process the conversion of genes to proteins. They even work as energy transducers, assisting in the conversion of food to energy.

What causes uric acid in the blood?

Uric acid is the end product of purines. It serves no biochemical function. Once uric acid is formed, it is usually eliminated from the body.

About one third of the uric acid normally produced in the body comes from food, with the remainder being produced through normal metabolism.

The final stages of purine metabolism include hypoxanthine to xanthine, and then from xanthine to uric acid. These are accomplished by the enzyme xanthine oxidase. Many gout patients take the xanthine oxidase inhibitor, allopurinol. This medication helps to prevent purines from ultimately metabolizing into uric acid.

Ovo-Lacto-Vegetarian Diet?

The dishes in this book represent an ovo-lacto-vegetarian diet. "Ovo," meaning eggs, and "lacto," meaning milk, are both allowed.

Why are the food lists in this book different from the food lists in the first Gout Hater's Cookbook?

Our first book, *Gout Hater's Cookbook, Recipes Lower in Purines and Lower in Fat*, is based on the *modified* purine diet, which allows a moderately small amount of meat and some foods relatively high in purines.

11

Book II is the perfect addition to the Gout Hater's collection. This book, which meets, as well as exceeds, the requirements of the modified purine diet in our first book, also complies with the restricted purine diet. It can therefore be used by patients on either regimen.

The recipes you will find in *Book II* feature a more detailed, albeit restricted, food list, on a delicious ovo-lacto- (eggs and milk allowed) vegetarian diet.

The recipes in *Book II* were put together in an effort to demonstrate just how delectably well you can eat, even on a restricted purine diet, while continually helping to lower your uric acid levels.

Why should we avoid Vitamin B-6 (Pyridoxine)?

There is no evidence to suggest that gout patients should avoid this supplement. However, decreasing the intake of B-6 to less than 2mg per day showed a dramatic improvement in patients with purine autism, significantly reducing purine related seizures. For this reason, we have chosen to avoid the supplement in our recipes.

In addition, too much vitamin B-6 can cause nerve injury as well as balance difficulties.

MSG (Monosodium Glutamate)

Although avoiding MSG is beneficial to your health, it can be quite difficult to detect its presence when checking labels for ingredients.

For instance, glutamates may not be specified when they are part of other ingredients, such as autolyzed yeast, hydrolyzed protein and yeast extract.

Always check your labels, especially those for instant soup mix, sauce mix, salad dressing, seasonings and stuffing mix and lowfat dairy products.

Other ingredient names to look out for include natural flavorings or flavors, yeast nutrient, "seasonings," textured protein, monosodium glutamate, and whey protein.

Xanthine

Xanthine is a purine base which appears in the metabolism of purines to uric acid. This compound is found in human muscle tissue, urine, blood and in some plants.

Included in the final stages of purine metabolism are those from hypoxanthine to xanthine, then from xanthine to uric acid.

Xanthine derivatives include caffeine, theobromine and theophylline. Theobromine and caffeine are found in chocolate, and both theobromine and theophylline as well as caffeine are found in tea.

Coffee, tea, chocolate, and cola drinks, as well as a multitude of other products, all contain xanthine or xanthine derivatives.

It is important to check ingredients for xanthine, xanthan gum or nonspecific vegetable gums. These ingredients appear often in dairy products such as yogurt, cream cheese and ice cream.

Always consult your physician before making any changes in your diet or eating habits.

Convert Your Own Recipes

Even on a restricted purine diet, eating can be fun, delicious and healthy.

As you work your way through our recipes, you will find a delicious assortment of recipes that can work for your diet.

However, this book is only the first step in your diet. Try using our recipes as a guide in changing some of your favorite high purine recipes into dishes that will work for you.

Many recipes which contain ingredients high in purines can be converted by substituting allowed foods. Try an experiment with some of your favorite past recipes.

Remove ingredients that are not allowed, and replace them with items that are acceptable to your diet.

For example, try replacing hamburger with the Veggie Burger recipe, page 64. Try replacing meatballs with the Falafel recipe, page 54.

Converting your past recipes into a dish that will comply with the restricted purine diet is a challenging, albeit rewarding, accomplishment. Each time you find you are able to successfully convert a recipe into one that complies with your diet, you will be one step closer towards changing the way you eat and live.

Congratulations on your successes!

• Does your recipe serve too many people or too few? You can change the amount of ingredients in a recipe by multiplying or dividing every ingredient by the same number.

Helpful Hints

Onions
When chopping onions for a recipe, try chopping several at a time in your food processor. Store them in your freezer in locking zipper bags for use at a later date.

Don't over-stuff the zipper bags. Place the bag on its side, and fill with just enough chopped onion to make a 1-inch layer. Place the bag in the freezer, also on its side. This way, small amounts can be easily broken off as needed.

Sautéing Your Foods
When sautéing foods, try using water instead of butter or margarine. This cuts down on the fat content of your dish. Simply place the ingredient to be sautéed in a non-stick skillet or saucepan, add water, and cook until the desired measure of doneness is reached and water is reduced. Add more water if necessary.

Lettuce
When preparing lettuce for a salad, always tear the lettuce by hand rather than cutting it with a knife. This will help prevent bruising.

Salt
When using salt, try including it in the preparation of the dish and not afterwards on individual servings. This will help reduce the overall amount of salt used.

Try substituting garlic powder for some, or all, of the salt as often as possible in these and other recipes. Your dish will be tastier and more healthy.

Coating your Ovenware
Try using a spray bottle filled with canola oil or olive oil to lightly mist your baking dish when cooking. "Pump" spray bottles can be found in the housewares section of your local department store.

Breakfast
Meals don't always have to be made from recipes with a great deal of preparation. For example, a breakfast of corn flakes, skim milk and fresh or dried fruit is simple, healthy and delicious.

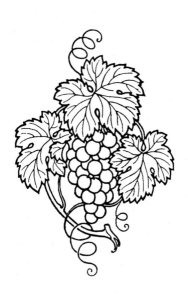

Breakfast

Spice Bars

1-1/2 teaspoons ginger, freshly grated
1-1/2 teaspoons pumpkin pie spice
3 egg whites
1 cup chopped raisins, dates or prunes
1/2 cup flour
1/2 cup chopped walnuts
1/2 teaspoon baking powder
1/3 cup sugar
2 teaspoons vanilla extract

Preheat oven to 350 degrees. Lightly coat a 9 x 5 x 3 bread pan with canola oil. Set aside.

Combine all ingredients in a large mixing bowl. Blend with electric mixer until thoroughly combined. Spread evenly in bottom of bread pan.

Bake for 20 minutes. Remove from oven and allow to cool. Cut crosswise. Makes six bars.

Rice Bars

1/2 cup chopped prunes
1/4 cup chopped dates
1/2 cup white rice flour
1/3 cup chopped pecans
1/2 cup cooked white rice
1/2 cup brown sugar
2 egg whites
1/2 teaspoon baking powder

Preheat oven to 350 degrees. Lightly coat a 9 x 5 x 3 bread pan with canola oil. Set aside.

Combine all ingredients in a medium mixing bowl. Blend with an electric mixer until thoroughly combined. Spread evenly in bottom of bread pan.

Bake for 20 minutes. Remove from oven, cool, and cut crosswise. Makes 6 bars.

Yogurt Honey Nut Bars

1-1/4 cup white rice flour
3 egg whites
1 teaspoon molasses
2 teaspoons honey
1 teaspoon vanilla extract
1/4 cup plain, nonfat yogurt (no xanthan gum)
1/2 cup pecans, chopped
1/2 cup walnuts, chopped
1/4 cup macadamia nuts, chopped
1/2 cup raisins or dates, chopped

Preheat oven to 350 degrees. Lightly coat a 9 x 5 x 3 bread pan with canola oil. Set aside.

Combine flour, egg whites, molasses, honey, vanilla extract and yogurt in a medium mixing bowl. Blend with an electric mixer until thoroughly combined.

Add nuts and raisins or dates. Stir well until evenly distributed. Spread evenly in bottom of bread pan.

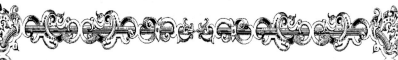

Bake for 30 minutes or until well browned and toothpick inserted in center comes out clean.

Allow to cool, then slice crosswise. Makes six bars.

Cherry Nut Bars

1/3 cup chopped walnuts
1/2 cup dried tart red cherries
3/4 cup white rice
1/2 cup white rice flour
1/2 teaspoon baking powder
2 egg whites
1 Tablespoon lemon juice
2 Tablespoons sugar

Preheat oven to 350 degrees. Lightly coat a 9 x 5 x 3 bread pan with canola oil. Set aside.

Combine all ingredients in a medium mixing bowl. Blend with an electric mixer until thoroughly combined, about 3 minutes. Spread evenly in bottom of bread pan. Bake

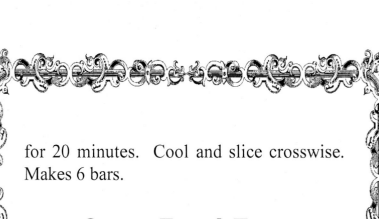

for 20 minutes. Cool and slice crosswise.
Makes 6 bars.

Orange French Toast

1/4 cup all purpose flour
1 teaspoon baking powder
1/8 teaspoon salt
3/4 cup orange juice
1/4 cup brown sugar
2 egg whites
1/2 teaspoon cinnamon
8 slices white bread

Combine all ingredients, except white bread,
in a large mixing bowl. Blend with a whisk
until smooth. Preheat a non-stick skillet.

Dip bread slices into mixture, turning to coat
evenly. Cook in skillet until lightly browned
on each side. Serve without syrup. Serves
four.

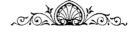

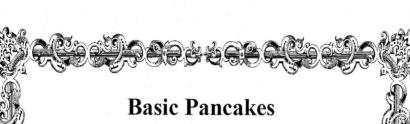

Basic Pancakes

2 egg whites
1 cup all purpose flour
1/2 teaspoon salt
1 teaspoon baking powder
3/4 cup skim milk
2 Tablespoons margarine, softened
2 Tablespoons sugar

Beat egg whites with an electric mixer until stiff. Set aside.

Combine remaining ingredients in a medium mixing bowl. Blend with electric mixer until a batter forms. Fold in egg whites with a whisk. Stir gently until blended.

Pour four inch circles of batter into a preheated, non-stick skillet. Flip pancakes when bubbles begin to appear throughout batter. Color should be light to rich brown. Serve warm with light syrup.
Makes one dozen.
Variation: Increase flour by 1/8 cup and add 1/2 cupblueberries to batter before cooking.

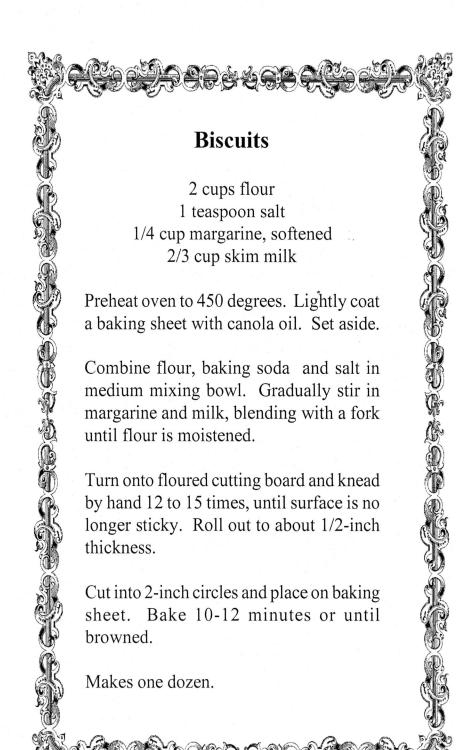

Biscuits

2 cups flour
1 teaspoon salt
1/4 cup margarine, softened
2/3 cup skim milk

Preheat oven to 450 degrees. Lightly coat a baking sheet with canola oil. Set aside.

Combine flour, baking soda and salt in medium mixing bowl. Gradually stir in margarine and milk, blending with a fork until flour is moistened.

Turn onto floured cutting board and knead by hand 12 to 15 times, until surface is no longer sticky. Roll out to about 1/2-inch thickness.

Cut into 2-inch circles and place on baking sheet. Bake 10-12 minutes or until browned.

Makes one dozen.

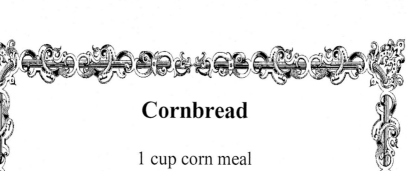

Cornbread

1 cup corn meal
1 cup flour
4 teaspoons baking powder
1/2 teaspoon salt
2 teaspoons sugar
1 cup milk
2 egg whites
1/3 cup canola oil

Preheat oven to 425 degrees. Lightly coat muffin tins with canola oil. Set aside.

Combine ingredients in a medium mixing bowl. Blend with an electric mixer until smooth, about 3 minutes. Pour into muffin tins. Bake for 18-20 minutes or until golden brown. Cool and serve.
Makes 1 dozen muffins.

Chili Pepper Cornbread

Add 1/2 cup chopped green chili peppers (seeds and pith removed) to cornbread recipe ingredients.

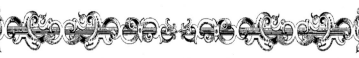

Denver Omelet

1/4 green bell pepper, chopped
1/4 red bell pepper, chopped
1 heaping Tablespoon finely chopped onion
1/4 cup water
1 egg
1 egg white
1/4 cup skim milk
1/3 cup grated cheese

Place peppers, onion and water in a preheated non-stick omelet pan (or 8-inch non-stick skillet). Sauté, stirring often, until water is reduced.

While peppers and onions are cooking, combine eggs and milk in a mixing bowl. Lightly beat with a whisk. Add cheese and stir until evenly coated. Once water has fully reduced, add egg mixture.

Cook; lifting edges continually with the corner of a spatula to allow excess liquid to reach pan surface. Gently flip after bottom is lightly browned and remainder is cooked enough to

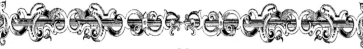

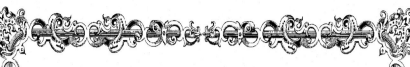

keep from breaking apart. Cook until lightly browned.

Rice Flour Pancakes

1-1/4 cup white rice flour
2 teaspoons baking powder
2 teaspoons sugar
1/2 teaspoon salt
1 cup skim milk
1 egg white

Combine all ingredients in a mixing bowl. Blend with an electric mixer until smooth. Cook on a pre-heated non-stick skillet, pouring about 1/8 cup per pancake.

Flip when bottom begins to brown and top appears to dry slightly, cooking about 3-4 minutes per side. Makes 8-10 four-inch pancakes.

Appetizers, Soups and Beverages

Cream of Celery Soup

6 stalks of celery
1 small onion
2 cups water
1 teaspoon salt
a pinch of pepper
2 Tablespoons flour
2 cups skim milk

Chop celery and onion. Combine in saucepan with water, salt and pepper. Bring to a boil and cook, stirring occasionally, about 15 minutes, until the celery and onion are transparent and water is reduced. Remove from heat and set aside.

Combine flour and milk, stirring with a fork until dissolved.

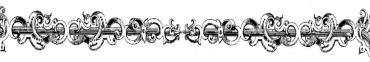

Add to celery mixture. Transfer to a blender and puree for about 30 seconds or until texture becomes smooth. Return to saucepan and cook, stirring frequently, until thickened to desired consistency. Remove from heat and serve immediately. Optional: garnish with chopped green onions or chopped celery. Serves four.

Vegetable Bouillon

2 quarts water
1 teaspoon salt
1 large onion, chopped
1 lb. carrots, peeled and sliced
5 stalks celery, chopped
6 oz. (one small can) tomato paste
1/4 teaspoon pepper
1 Tablespoon lemon juice
1/4 teaspoon pepper

Combine ingredients in a large pot. Bring to a boil. Reduce heat and cover. Continue cooking, stirring occasionally, for about 30 minutes, until vegetables are cooked. Allow to cool.

Drain and save liquid for vegetable

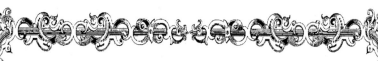

bouillon. Refrigerate until ready for use. Vegetables may be saved and used for a side dish.

Tomato Soup

2 cups tomato juice
2 cups vegetable bouillon
Tabasco sauce

Combine tomato sauce and bouillon in saucepan. Heat, stirring occasionally. Add Tabasco sauce to taste and serve. Serves four. Variation: Add tomato chunks and vegetables from vegetable bouillon.

Beet Soup

4 medium beets, peeled and chopped
(tops discarded)
2-1/2 cups water
1/2 cup onions, chopped
1 cup carrots, peeled and sliced
1 Tablespoon lemon juice
1 Tablespoon sugar
2 Tablespoons vinegar

Combine ingredients in a large saucepan. Bring to a boil. Reduce heat and cover,

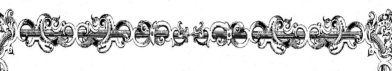

cooking for about 15 minutes. Serve topped with a spoonful of nonfat yogurt (optional). Serves 4.

Matzoh Ball Soup

Matzoh balls:
3/4 cup matzoh meal
4 egg whites
3 Tablespoons margarine, softened
3 Tablespoons water
1/2 teaspoon salt
1/2 teaspoon garlic powder

Soup:
3 quarts water
6 green onions, chopped
3 stalks celery, chopped
4 carrots, peeled and chopped
2 teaspoons minced garlic
2 teaspoons salt

Combine matzoh ball ingredients in a mixing bowl. Stir with fork until well blended. Set aside, chilling in refrigerator for at least 30 minutes (Chilling overnight is actually better; the matzoh balls will come out feathery).

Combine soup ingredients in a large pot. Bring to a boil and reduce heat. Cover and simmer, cooking while matzoh balls are being made.

To make matzoh balls: In another pot, bring 3 quarts of water to a boil. While water is heating, remove matzoh meal dough from refrigerator.

Wet hands with water, then form dough into one-inch balls (Makes about 18). Once water has come to a boil, reduce heat to simmer.

Drop balls into gently boiling water. Cover and simmer for about 35 minutes or until cooked throughout. Remove matzoh balls from water with slotted spoon; add to soup. Serves 4-6.

Egg Drop Soup

1 quart water
6 chopped green onions
2 teaspoons minced garlic
1 Tablespoon dried chopped onion
1/2 teaspoon salt
1/8 teaspoon pepper
1/2 teaspoon freshly ground ginger
2 egg whites

Combine all ingredients except egg in a medium sauce pan. Bring to a boil, cooking about 5 minutes. In a small mixing bowl, stir egg whites briefly with a whisk. Then, while stirring soup briskly with whisk, add egg whites to soup.

Stir constantly, cooking for about 30 seconds, until egg is cooked, and serve.

Serves four.

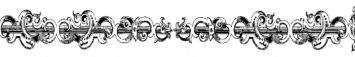

Cheese Soup

1 medium onion, finely chopped
1-1/2 cups water
1/2 teaspoon paprika
1 teaspoon salt
1-1/2 teaspoons dijon mustard
1/4 teaspoon pepper
3 Tablespoons tomato paste
3 cups skim milk
2 Tablespoons cornstarch
4 ounces reduced fat sharp cheddar cheese

In medium saucepan, combine onion, 1/2 cup water, paprika, salt, mustard and pepper. Sauté, stirring frequently, until liquid is reduced. Add remaining water, tomato paste and 2 1/2 cups milk. Heat, stirring occasionally, to boiling point. Reduce heat and simmer.

Combine remaining milk and cornstarch in a small mixing bowl. Blend with a fork until smooth, then add to saucepan. Add cheese and stir. Return to a boil, then reduce heat and cook, stirring frequently, until cheese is melted and soup is slightly thickened, about 20 to 25 minutes.Serve immediately with toasted bread. Serves four.

Vegetable Salad

2/3 cup celery, chopped
1/2 cup carrots, grated
1 cup corn, cut fresh from cob
1/3 cup Mayonnaise (see page 82)
2 Tablespoons onion, finely chopped
1/4 cup parmesan cheese, grated
1 Tablespoon vinegar

Place celery, carrots and corn in mixing bowl. Set aside. Combine remaining ingredients in blender and mix well. Pour over vegetables, folding until evenly coated. Cover and chill. Fold again before serving.

Serves 2-3.

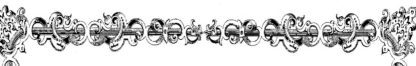

Cucumber Dill Salad

1 large cucumber
1 medium tomato
1/2 medium onion
2 teaspoons dill weed
1 oz. vinegar
1/4 cup canola oil

Peel, slice and quarter cucumber. Place in mixing bowl. Chop tomato and add. Thinly slice onion, not in rings, and add. Add remaining ingredients. Fold until vinegar and oil are blended and all is evenly coated. Set aside to marinate in refrigerator for 10-15 minutes. Fold again before serving.

Serves two.

Cheese Salad

2 Tablespoons vinegar
4 Tablespoons oil
2 Tablespoons coarse Dijon mustard
3 cloves garlic, pressed
3 Tablespoons onion, finely chopped
2 ounces low sodium Swiss cheese
2 ounces reduced fat sharp cheddar
1/3 cup green olives with pimiento,
lightly chopped
1/2 bell pepper, finely chopped
1 boiled egg, chopped, yolk discarded

Combine vinegar, oil, mustard, garlic, and onion in a small mixing bowl. Stir well. Set aside for at least 15 minutes. This will give the ingredients a chance to blend.

Cut cheese into small, bite size cubes. Place in medium mixing bowl. Add olives, peppers, chopped egg white and dressing. Toss well and serve.
Serves four.

Tip: This salad is even better if chilled overnight, after the cheese has had a chance to absorb all of the flavors.

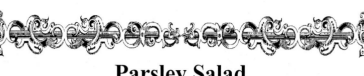

Parsley Salad

1 bunch fresh parsley, chopped
20 fresh mint leaves, chopped
2 cups romaine lettuce leaves, torn to bite
size pieces
1 medium tomato, cut into wedges
lemon dressing (see page 84)

Combine ingredients in salad bowl. Toss until all are evenly coated and serve.
Serves four.

Note: This salad has a slightly bitter taste. This can be altered, if preferred, by adding a teaspoon of sugar to the dressing, reducing the amount of parsley, or increasing the amount of romaine lettuce.

Bell Pepper Salad

1 bell pepper
1/3 cup Italian dressing (see recipe, page 85)

Remove seeds and pith from pepper. Slice thinly. Toss in dressing. Serve chilled.
Serves two.

Broccoli Salad

1 stalk of broccoli
2 fresh cobs of corn
1/2 cup celery, finely chopped
Parmesan Dressing (see page 83, ·

Break broccoli head into small pieces and place in mixing bowl. Peel and chop stem. Add to bowl.

Cut corn from cobs and add. Add celery. Fold in dressing and toss until evenly coated. Serve chilled. Serves four.

Green Bean Salad

1-1/2 cups green beans, cooked
1/3 cup Italian dressing (see recipe, page 85)

Combine beans with dressing. Toss until evenly coated; serve.
Serves two.

Tips: This can be kept in the refrigerator for a few days, but the taste is better when served

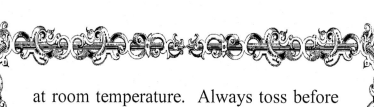

at room temperature. Always toss before serving.

Egg Salad

1 stalk celery, finely chopped celery
3 eggs, boiled (discard two yolks)
2 heaping Tablespoons onion, finely chopped
1/8 teaspoon paprika
1/4 teaspoon garlic powder
1/8 teaspoon pepper
1/8 teaspoon salt
2 Tablespoons plain, nonfat yogurt (no xanthan gum) or mayonnaise (page 82)
4 slices French bread

Combine ingredients in a medium mixing bowl (don't forget to discard two of the egg yolks). Stir with a spoon until blended. Serve over thinly sliced, toasted French bread.

Serves two.

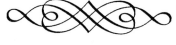

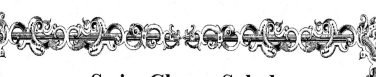

Swiss Cheese Salad

1/4 pound reduced fat Swiss cheese, cut into
thin slices
3 cups endive lettuce, cut into bite size
pieces
Croutons (see page 42)
Honey Mustard Dressing (see page 85)

Cut cheese slices into 1-inch squares. Place in
salad bowl with lettuce. Add croutons and
dressing. Toss and serve. Serves four.

Egg Salad Wedges

Three rounds of pita bread, cut into wedges
One egg salad recipe (see page 40)

Place a portion of egg salad on the pointed end
of each pita wedge, leaving enough room on
rounded end for easy handling with fingers.
Makes 18-24.

Croutons

1 Tablespoon margarine
2 cups of cubes cut from white, French
or Italian bread
1 teaspoon parmesan cheese, grated
1/2 teaspoon garlic powder

Heat margarine in skillet. After it begins to sizzle, toss in bread. Flip with spatula until margarine is distributed.

Sprinkle one half of parmesan and one half of garlic powder over bread. Toss with spatula, then sprinkle remaining parmesan and garlic.

Toss frequently until browned. Cool and add to salad.

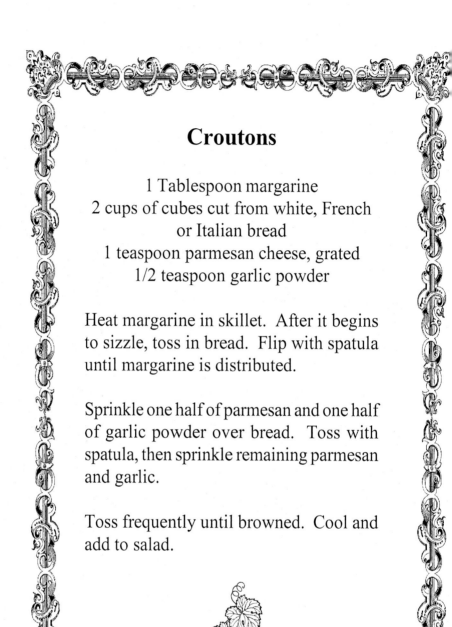

Roasted Cheese

1 cup low-fat ricotta cheese (no xanthan gum)
1 egg white
1 sprig rosemary, chopped
6 sprigs parsley, chopped
1/4 teaspoon powdered cumin
6 cloves garlic, pressed
20 grape leaves
olive oil

Preheat oven at 350 degrees. Lightly coat a cookie sheet with olive oil. Set aside.

In a medium mixing bowl, combine ricotta, egg, rosemary, parsley, cumin and garlic. Blend with electric mixer until thoroughly combined. Place one teaspoon of this mixture in the center of each grape leaf. Top with two drops olive oil.

Wrap by folding upward and overlapping edges of leaves over cheese. Hold with toothpicks.

Bake for 20 minutes. Serve warm or at room temperature.

Makes twenty.

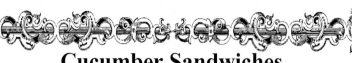

Cucumber Sandwiches

1 large seedless cucumber
6 slices white bread, toasted
plain, nonfat yogurt (no xanthan gum)
dill weed

Peel cucumber. Remove ends and slice thinly using the slicing portion of a cheese grater. Pat slices dry and set aside.

With a small cookie cutter (small enough to fit inside the circumference of cucumber slices), cut shapes in bread. You should be able to get six shapes per piece of bread. Lay out bread shapes on serving dish. Save remaining bread for another recipe, such as croutons.

Cut out the same shapes in the cucumber slices. (Save remaining cucumber for another recipe, such as cucumber salad. Set the cucumber shapes on top of the bread shapes. Top each cucumber shape with a small dab of yogurt and a light sprinkle of dill weed.

Makes about 3 dozen

Taco Melt Wedges

4 flour tortillas, 8-inch
1 cup reduced fat cheese, grated
1/2 green bell pepper, chopped
1/2 chili pepper, chopped
2 heaping Tablespoons onion, finely chopped

Separate cheese, both kinds of peppers and onion into equal halves. On each of two tortillas, evenly sprinkle cheese, peppers and onion. Top with remaining tortillas.

Place each tortilla "sandwich" in preheated non-stick skillet until lightly browned and cheese is melted. Flip and lightly brown on reverse side.

Remove from skillet and place on cutting board. Cut into eighths with a butcher knife by gently rocking back and forth until fully cut.
Makes 16 wedges (eight servings).

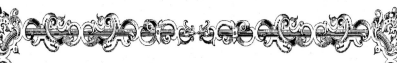

Lemon Ginger Tea

1 cubic inch chunk of fresh ginger
1 qt. water
3 teaspoons lemon juice

Peel and chop ginger. Place in a tea ball and set aside. Bring water to a boil. Transfer to a teapot, adding lemon juice and tea ball. Steep 5-7 minutes and serve. May be sweetened with honey if desired.

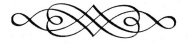

Cranberry Tea

2 cups water
2 cups cranberry juice
1 cinnamon stick

Combine ingredients in a medium saucepan. Bring to a boil, cover and steep 2-3 minutes. Remove cinnamon and serve.
Makes 4 cups.

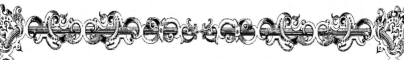

Berry Yogurt Freeze

1/2 cup plain, nonfat yogurt (no xanthan gum)
1/2 cup orange juice
1/2 cup berries
1/2 cup ice

Combine all ingredients in a blender and puree until smooth. This is a delightful summer cooler.
Serves two.

Pineapple Lime Fizz

1-1/4 lemon-lime soda
1-2/3 cups pineapple juice
1 oz. lime juice

Combine and serve. Makes a great punch.
Serves two.

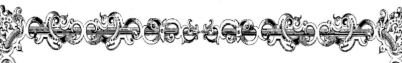

Cranberry Water

2 cups water
1-1/3 cup cranberry juice

Combine and serve.

Serves two.

Orange Lime Shake

1/3 cup lime juice
1/2 cup orange juice
1/2 cup water
4 Tablespoons sugar
1 cup ice

Combine ingredients in blender. Mix for about one minute or until smooth and serve.

Serves two.

Virgin Margarita

1/3 cup lime juice
1 cup water
4 Tablespoons sugar
1 cup ice

Combine all ingredients in blender. Mix for about one minute or until smooth.

Serves two.

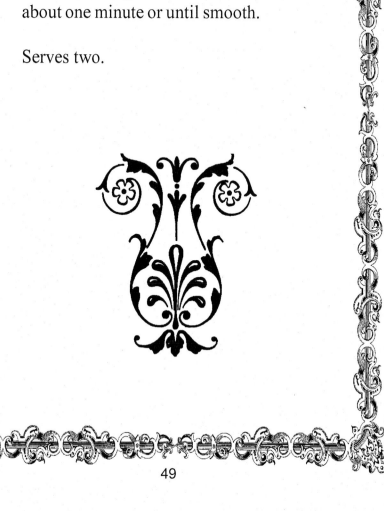

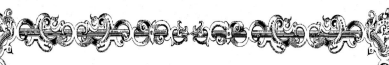

Main Dishes

Onion Broccoli Quiche

1 9-inch pie crust
1 egg
2 egg whites
1/2 cup reduced fat grated Swiss cheese
1/2 cup reduced fat grated cheddar cheese
1/2 cup onion, finely chopped
2 cups broccoli, chopped, tops only
3 cloves garlic, pressed
1/2 cup plain, nonfat yogurt (no xanthan gum)
1/8 teaspoon pepper

Preheat oven to 375 degrees. Prick holes in pie crust with a fork. Set aside.

Combine egg and egg whites in a medium mixing bowl. Stir with a whisk until blended. Add remaining ingredients, stirring with fork until evenly distributed.

Pour into pie crust. Bake for 45 minutes or until golden brown. Can be served warm or chilled. Serves eight.

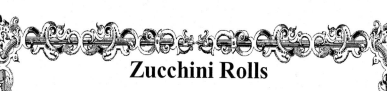

Zucchini Rolls

8 lasagna noodles (about 1/2 pound)
1 egg white, lightly beaten
3 cloves garlic, pressed
1/4 cup onions, chopped
1/8 teaspoon pepper
1/2 teaspoon dried oregano
32 oz. spaghetti sauce
1 zucchini squash, chopped
1-1/8 cups part skim mozzarella, grated

Prepare lasagna noodles according to package directions. While noodles are cooking, egg white, garlic, onions, pepper, oregano and zucchini in mixing bowl. Stir until ingredients are well distributed.

Preheat oven to 350 degrees. Lightly coat a 15 x 11 x 2 inch baking dish with olive oil. Set aside.

Once noodles have cooked, drain, rinse and lay out. On each noodle, spread a layer of zucchini mixture, about three to four heaping teaspoonsful. Over the zucchini, spread a light layer of sauce.

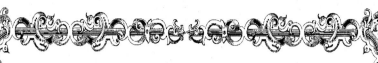

Sprinkle grated mozzarella over sauce, about 1/8 cup per noodle.

Roll each noodle and place in baking dish, folded side down. Once all rolls have been placed into the baking dish, cover with remaining sauce.

Cover dish with foil and bake 45 minutes. Makes 8 rolls.

Baked Polenta

2 cups water
2 cups skim milk
2 teaspoons salt
1 teaspoon sugar
2 pinches ground cinnamon
1 cup finely ground corn meal
1-1/4 cup dried cherries
3 small boxes (3/4 cup) raisins
1 Tablespoon margarine

Preheat oven to 350 degrees. Lightly coat a 2 quart casserole dish with canola oil. Set aside.

Combine water, milk, salt and sugar in a large saucepan. Heat to the boiling point, then reduce heat to medium. Add cornmeal and continue to cook for about one minute, stirring frequently.

Stir in cherries and raisins. Transfer to the casserole dish. Flake the margarine over the surface of the cornmeal mixture.

Bake 30 minutes or until surface becomes golden brown. Serves four.

Variations: Combine or substitute cherries and raisins with chopped or sliced apples, pears or prunes.

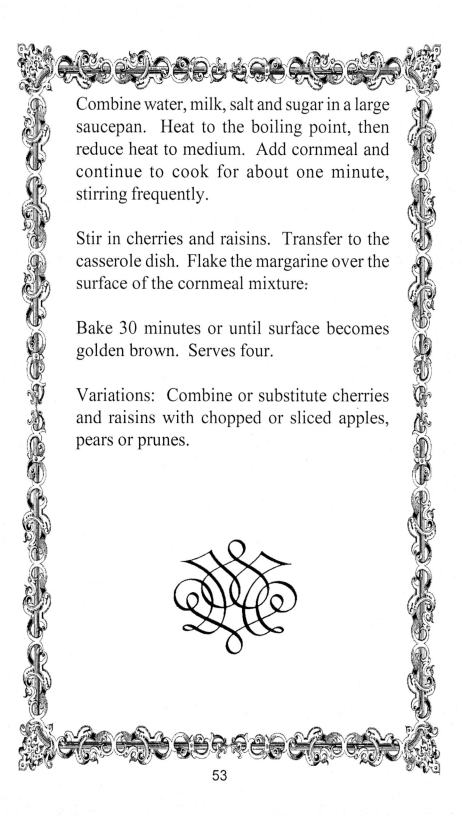

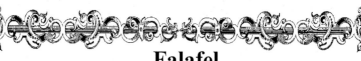

Falafel

1 cup onion, finely chopped
1/2 cup water
1 large potato, cooked and peeled
1 teaspoon powdered cumin
1 teaspoon dried (or 8 sprigs fresh) chopped
parsley
1 teaspoon salt
1/2 teaspoon pepper
2 egg whites
1/2 cup flour
5 cloves garlic, pressed
1 teaspoon baking soda

Cook onion in 1/2 cup water in a small sauce pan for about 15 minutes or until onion is transparent and water is reduced. Set aside to cool.

Mash potato. Place in a large mixing bowl. Add cooled onion and remaining ingredients. Blend with whisk until thoroughly combined. Shape into 1-inch balls.

Pre-heat a non-stick skillet with 1 Tablespoon canola oil. Cook falafel balls

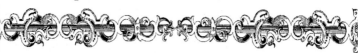

in skillet, turning as needed, until browned.

Serve warm or chilled. Serves four.

Olive and Tomato Pasta

1/2 pound pasta
1 tomato, medium to large
1/2 cup black olives
2 cloves garlic, pressed
2 Tablespoons olive oil

Prepare pasta according to package directions. While pasta is cooking, add tomato to boiling water for about thirty seconds. Remove tomato and cool under running water. Remove skin and chop. Place into preheated saucepan with olives, garlic and 1 Tablespoon of olive oil. Sauté, stirring frequently, until heated.

Toss into cooked pasta with remaining olive oil.

Serves two.

Stuffed Tomatoes

2 large, ripe tomatoes
4 large romaine lettuce leaves
1 cup small pasta, cooked and chilled
1 egg, boiled, yolk discarded
1-1/2 teaspoons Dijon mustard
1 teaspoon paprika
1/8 teaspoon pepper˒
1/2 cup plain, nonfat yogurt (no xanthan gum)
3 teaspoons dried parsley flakes
1/4 teaspoon garlic powder
1/4 teaspoon salt

Slice top off and hollow out each tomato. Drain excess liquid from hollowed tomatoes and place on serving dish over romaine leaves. Set aside.

Chop remaining tomato and place in mixing bowl. Chop egg white and add to bowl. Add remaining ingredients to bowl. Stir with spoon until blended.

Spoon into tomatoes. Any remaining filling may be spooned onto romaine leaves around tomatoes. Sprinkle with parsley flakes or paprika. Serves two.

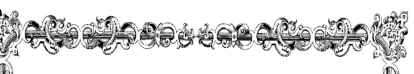

Eggplant Pasta
with Lemon Pepper

1/2 pound pasta
2 cups eggplant, peeled and diced
1/4 cup onions, chopped
1/2 cup water
1 teaspoon dried parsley
1/2 teaspoon pepper
1 cup skim milk
1/2 teaspoon salt
1 Tablespoon cornstarch
2 Tablespoons lemon juice

Prepare pasta according to package directions. While pasta is cooking, com-bine eggplant, onion, water, parsley and pepper in a medium saucepan. Sauté until water is reduced and onions are transparent.

Combine milk, salt and cornstarch, stirring until smooth. Add to saucepan. Cook until thickened, stirring often. Add lemon juice and cook again until thickened. Fold into cooked pasta and serve.
Serves two.

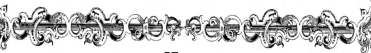

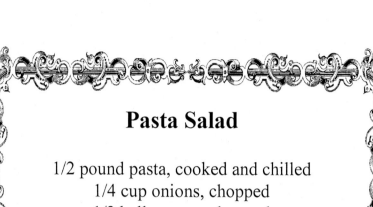

Pasta Salad

1/2 pound pasta, cooked and chilled
1/4 cup onions, chopped
1/2 bell pepper, chopped
1/2 cup black olives, chopped (watch for
additives)
2 Tablespoons vinegar.
4 Tablespoons olive or canola oil
1/8 teaspoon pepper
1/2 teaspoon dried parsley flakes

Combine ingredients in a large mixing bowl.
Fold until evenly distributed. Serve chilled
or at room temperature.

Serves two.

**People in history said to have suffered from
gout include most of the Roman emperors,
Martin Luther, Henry VIII, John Calvin,
Francis Bacon, Sir Isaac Newton and
Benjamin Franklin.**

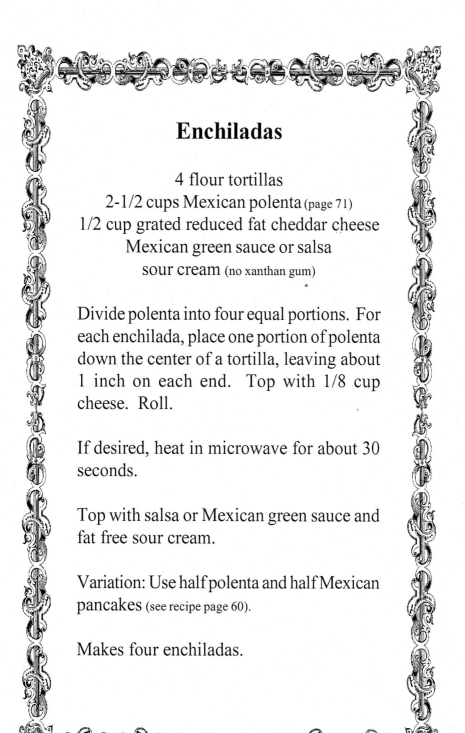

Enchiladas

4 flour tortillas
2-1/2 cups Mexican polenta (page 71)
1/2 cup grated reduced fat cheddar cheese
Mexican green sauce or salsa
sour cream (no xanthan gum)

Divide polenta into four equal portions. For each enchilada, place one portion of polenta down the center of a tortilla, leaving about 1 inch on each end. Top with 1/8 cup cheese. Roll.

If desired, heat in microwave for about 30 seconds.

Top with salsa or Mexican green sauce and fat free sour cream.

Variation: Use half polenta and half Mexican pancakes (see recipe page 60).

Makes four enchiladas.

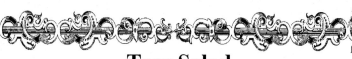

Taco Salad

corn chips
Mexican pancake, cut into chunks
lettuce, finely torn
reduced fat cheddar cheese, grated
fresh tomato, chopped
salsa

For each serving of taco salad, place from bottom to top a layer of corn chips, Mexican pancake chunks, finely torn lettuce, 1/8 cup grated cheese, chopped tomato and salsa.

Mexican Pancakes

1-3/4 cup flour
1 teaspoon baking powder
2 egg whites
1 cup salsa
3/4 cup skim milk
1/4 cup margarine, softened

Combine dry ingredients in medium mixing bowl. Add remaining ingredients, blending with mixer until batter is formed.

Pour batter into pre-heated, non-stick skillet. Cook until bubbles begin to appear and bottom browns, then flip and cook on other side.

These can be eaten as pancakes or cut into pieces and used in tacos, enchiladas, etc.

Serves four.

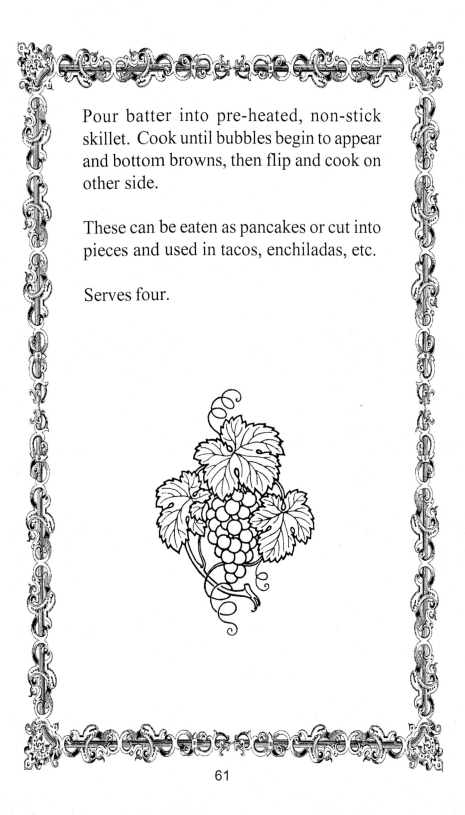

Fajitas

2 bell peppers
1 small onion
3/4 cup water
4 flour tortillas
1/2 cup reduced fat cheese, grated
(cheddar or Monterey Jack)

Remove top and pith from peppers. Slice thinly and set aside. Thinly slice or chop onion.

Place onion, peppers and 1/4 cup water in a pre-heated non-stick skillet. Cook about 5 minutes, stirring frequently, until water is reduced. After peppers and onions begin to brown, stir in remaining water.

Continue cooking. Water will turn brown and begin to evaporate. Stir well to coat peppers and onions. Remove from heat.

Place 1/4 of mixture over each of the flour tortillas and top with 1/8 cup cheese.

Makes four fajitas.

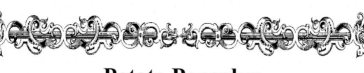

Potato Pancakes

3 cups potatoes, cooked and chopped
4 egg whites
3 Tablespoons flour
1 teaspoon salt
1/3 cup finely chopped onions
1 teaspoon parsley

Mash potatoes with masher. Combine with remaining ingredients in a medium mixing bowl.

Blend with mixer for about two minutes. (It's all right if there are lumps.)

Preheat a non-stick skillet. Lightly mist with canola oil. For each potato pancake, measure one heaping Tablespoon of "batter," cooking two to three minutes per side until well-browned. Lightly press down with spatula while cooking.

Serves four.

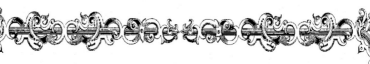

Veggie Burgers

1 cup cooked rice
2-1/2 to 3 cups chopped eggplant
1 1/2 cups water
6 cloves garlic, pressed
1/2 cup onion, finely chopped
1 teaspoon fresh parsley, chopped
1 large tomato, chopped
1/8 teaspoon pepper
1 Tablespoon oregano
1/8 teaspoon paprika
4 heaping Tablespoons parmesan
3 egg whites
1 cup flour

Combine rice, eggplant, water, garlic, onion, pepper, oregano, parsley and tomato and spices in a medium saucepan. Cook on high, stirring often, until water is absorbed. Remove from heat and allow to cool for 10-15 minutes.

Place in a large mixing bowl. Blend with electric mixer, gradually adding in parmesan, eggs and flour. Consistency will resemble chunky pancake batter.

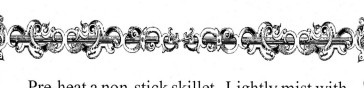

Pre-heat a non-stick skillet. Lightly mist with canola oil and drop in mixture. Use about 3 tablespoons of batter for each burger.

Flatten burgers slightly with spatula. Sprinkle tops lightly with additional parmesan. Cook 2 to 3 minutes, or until browned, on each side.

Serve over hamburger buns with lettuce, tomato and pickle. This is also good served simply over rice.
Makes 8 to 10 burgers.

Spaghetti Squash

one spaghetti squash
32 ounces (4 cups) spaghetti sauce
grated parmesan cheese

Preheat oven at 425 degrees. Cut squash in half and remove seeds. Place squash in oven-proof pan, "open bowl" side upward. Pour 2 cups of spaghetti sauce into opening of each half. Cover with foil and roast for 1-1/2 hours. Remove from oven and lightly lift out strands of squash onto a serving dish. Top with grated parmesan. Serves two.

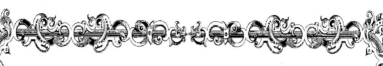

Pizza

pizza sauce (see below or page 76)
4 cups flour
4 teaspoons baking powder
1-1/2 teaspoons salt
2 teaspoons sugar
1/2 cup skim milk (warmed 20 sec. in microwave)
1/2 cup warm water
2 egg whites
2 Tablespoons olive oil
4 ounces part skim mozzarella, grated
1/2 cup onion, chopped
1/2 bell pepper, chopped
1/3 cup sliced olives, black or green
oregano

Prepare pizza sauce according to recipe. Set aside. Preheat oven to 375 degrees. Lightly coat a cookie sheet with olive oil. Set aside.

Combine flour, baking powder, salt, sugar, milk, water, egg whites and olive oil in large mixing bowl. Knead with floured hands until dough loses its sticky feel. Place on flat surface, sprinkle with

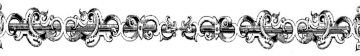

additional flour and roll thin.

Place pizza dough in cookie sheet, stretching lightly with fingers, if needed, until the dough reaches the edges of the cookie sheet.

Brush surface of dough with additional olive oil. spread sauce, then sprinkle cheese, onions, peppers and olives. Top with oregano.

Bake for 25 to 30 minutes or until dough both dough and cheese are brown. Serves four.

Pizza Sauce

5 medium tomatoes
2 quarts water
1-1/2 cups onions, chopped
4 cloves garlic, pressed
1 teaspoon oregano
1/2 teaspoon basil
2 teaspoons sugar
1 teaspoon lemon juice
1 teaspoon dried parsley
1/2 teaspoon salt

Bring water to boil in a large pot. Remove tops from tomatoes, discarding the tops. Add the tomatoes to the pot. Continue boiling about 5 minutes. Remove tomatoes with a slotted spoon and place in colander. Cool in colander under running water.

While tomatoes are cooling, add remaining ingredients to pot. Bring to a boil, then reduce heat and simmer.

Once tomatoes have cooled, remove their skins and discard. Return tomatoes to pot. Return to a boil. Continue cooking, stirring occasionally, until water is reduced and sauce thickens to desired consistency, about 45 to 60 minutes. Makes about 1-1/2 cups.

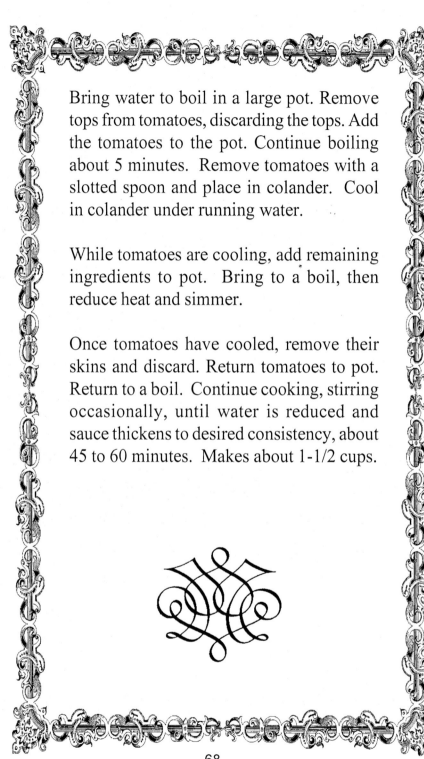

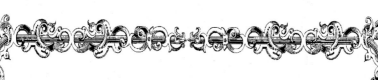

Sides and Sauces

Mint Carrots

1 lb. peeled baby carrots
6 dozen fresh mint leaves, chopped
2 cups water
1 Tablespoon ground arrowroot
4 teaspoons lemon juice
1 1/2 Tablespoons brown sugar

Combine ingredients in a medium saucepan.

Bring to a boil. Cover and simmer, stirring occasionally, for about 10 minutes.

Uncover and cook, stirring occasionally, until liquid is reduced to a glaze (about 35 minutes). Cool about 10 minutes and stir.

Serves four.

Roasted Potatoes

1-1/2 lb. potatoes
3/4 cup fresh ground romano or parmesan
1 teaspoon dried oregano
Garlic Sauce (see recipe, page 77)

Preheat oven to 350 degrees. Lightly coat an 8 x 8 x 2 baking dish with olive oil. Set aside.

Peel potatoes and cut into bite-sized chunks (about 4 cups). Place in bottom of cooking dish. Sprinkle cheese evenly over potatoes, then sprinkle oregano evenly over cheese.

Bake covered for 30 minutes. Remove cover, and continue baking for about 15 minutes, or until surface has browned.

Check for doneness by inserting fork into a piece near the center of baking dish.

Remove from oven and serve covered with garlic sauce.

Serves four.

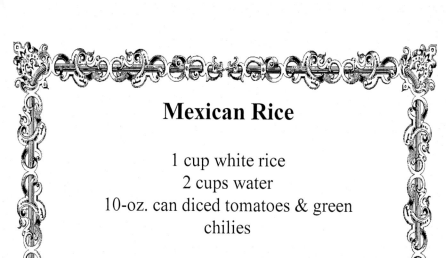

Mexican Rice

1 cup white rice
2 cups water
10-oz. can diced tomatoes & green
chilies

Combine ingredients in a saucepan. Bring to a boil, uncovered. Cook for one minute.

Stir, cover and reduce heat, simmering for about 20 minutes. Do not remove cover while simmering. Do not stir.

Remove from heat and cool, still covered, for 5 minutes; uncover and serve.
Makes 3 cups.

Mexican Polenta

3/4 cup fine cornmeal
1-1/2 cup Mexican Salsa (see recipe, page 79)
1 egg white
1/2 cup reduced fat cheddar cheese,
grated
2 cups water

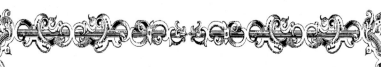

Combine ingredients, stirring well. Place in saucepan. Cook, stirring frequentlyuntil water is reduced and thickness resembles that of oatmeal. Serve hot.

Makes four servings.

Broccoli with Plum Sauce

4 stalks broccoli, peeled and chopped
1/2 cup plum preserves or jelly
2 Tablespoon vinegar
2 teaspoons dried minced onion
1 teaspoon dried minced garlic
1 teaspoon freshly ground ginger

Steam broccoli briefly in a food steamer (or in a covered pot with one quart water) until just tender but still crispy, about 10 minutes. Set aside.

Combine remaining ingredients in sauce pan and heat, stirring constantly, cooking about five minutes. Add broccoli and fold until coated.

Serves four.

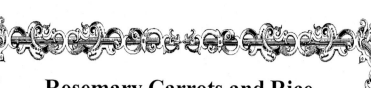

Rosemary Carrots and Rice

2 cups water
2 sprigs fresh rosemary, chopped
1/8 teaspoon salt
1/2 lb. baby carrots
2 dozen fresh mint leaves, chopped
1/2 cup rice

In medium saucepan, combine all ingredients except rice. Bring to a boil, cooking about 10 minutes until carrots are tender. Stir in rice, cover and simmer for 20 minutes. Remove from heat for about 5 minutes, allowing to cool and remaining liquid to be absorbed.

Serves four.

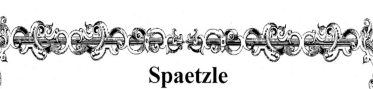

Spaetzle
(Little Dumplings)

3 cups flour
1/2 teaspoon salt
3 egg whites
1 cup water

Combine ingredients in medium mixing bowl, stirring with a fork until thoroughly blended. Chill for 20 minutes.

Boil 3 quarts water (lightly salted if desired). Drop dumplings by small pieces, either through potato press or by placing a small amount on cutting board and cutting and dragging off small pieces (about the size of two peas) into boiling water.

Cook for about three minutes, until dough has had a chance to drop to the bottom and return to the top.

Remove from boiling water with a slotted spoon and place in colander. Continue cooking spaeztle until dough supply has been used. Serve as a side or main dish, with margarine or sauce.

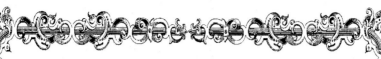

Rice Pilaf

2 cups rice
1 cup vermicelli
1 Tablespoon canola oil
2 teaspoon salt
1/2 teaspoon garlic powder
1/2 teaspoon onion powder
2-3/4 cups water

Combine all ingredients, except water, in saucepan. Sauté, stirring constantly, until rice and vermicelli are browned. Add water, bring to a boil, stir and cover.

Reduce heat and simmer for 20 minutes. Remove from heat and let sit, covered, for 10 minutes. Uncover and serve. Serves four.

Broccoli Cole Slaw

2 cups broccoli, finely chopped or julienne
1/2 cup grated carrots
1 stalk finely chopped celery
1/2 cup plain, nonfat yogurt (no xanthan gum)

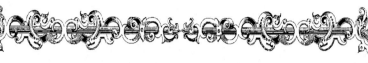

2 teaspoons vinegar
2 teaspoons sugar
1/8 teaspoon pepper

Combine ingredients in mixing bowl. Stir until well distributed.

Serves four.

Quick Pizza Sauce

2 6-ounce cans tomato paste
2 cups water
1-1/2 cups onions, chopped
1/2 Tablespoon garlic powder
1/2 teaspoon basil
2 teaspoons sugar
1 teaspoon lemon juice
1/2 teaspoon salt
1 teaspoon dried chopped parsley

Combine ingredients in a large pot. Bring to a boil. Cook about 10 minutes, or until desired consistency is reached. Stir constantly to prevent sticking or splattering.

Makes about 3 cups, enough for 2 pizzas.

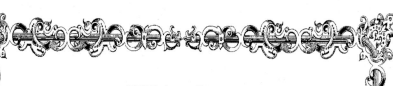

White Sauce

1 cup skim milk
1-1/2 Tablespoons flour
1/2 teaspoon salt
a pinch of dried chopped parsley
1 sprinkle pepper

Blend ingredients with a fork until smooth. Heat in a small saucepan, stirring constantly, until sauce thickens to desired consistency.

Garlic Sauce

1 cup milk
1-1/2 Tablespoons flour
1/4 teaspoon salt
3 cloves garlic, pressed
2 sprinkles pepper

Blend milk and flour with fork until smooth. Combine with remaining ingredients in small saucepan. Heat, stirring constantly, until sauce thickens to desired consistency.

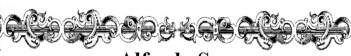

Alfredo Sauce

2 cups skim milk
2 teaspoons cornstarch
3 cloves garlic, pressed
1/2 teaspoon onion powder
1 teaspoons dried chopped parsley
1/2 teaspoon oregano
2 sprinkles pepper.
1/2 teaspoon salt

Combine milk and cornstarch, stirring with fork until blended. Place in saucepan with remaining ingredients. Cook over medium heat, stirring constantly, until sauce thickens. Serve over pasta or vegetables.

Light Curry Sauce

1 teaspoon sugar
1 teaspoon lemon juice
1 cup milk
1/4 teaspoon salt
1 Tablespoon cornstarch
1/2 teaspoon curry powder

Combine ingredients, stirring with a fork until smooth. Place in a small saucepan.

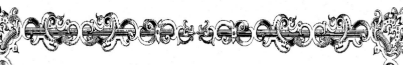

Heat to boiling, stirring frequently. Reduce heat and continue cooking, stirring frequently, until thickened. Serve over rice or vegetables.

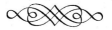

Mexican Salsa

one 14-oz. can stewed tomatoes in juice
2 oz. peeled & diced green chilies
(1 oz. for mild)
3 jalopenos, chopped
(reduce to 1 or zero for mild)
juice of one lime
1/2 medium white onion, chopped
1/2 teaspoon garlic powder
1 teaspoon sugar

Drain tomato juice into a mixing bowl. Chop tomatoes and add to bowl. Add remaining ingredients. Stir and let sit for 20 minutes. Serve with chips or fresh vegetables.

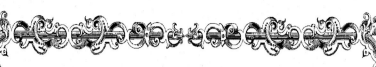

Mexican Green Sauce

2 oz. green chilies, chopped
1 Tablespoon vinegar
1/2 cup water
1/2 teaspoon garlic
2 teaspoons dried chopped onion
1 teaspoon flour
1-1/2 teaspoons sugar

Combine ingredients and puree in blender. Place in a small saucepan. Bring to a boil, stirring constantly, until thickened (consistency should be similar to thick gravy). Cool and serve.

Homemade Margarine

1/2 cup butter, softened
1/2 cup canola oil

Combine in blender. Blend for about 30 seconds. Transfer to airtight container and refrigerate.

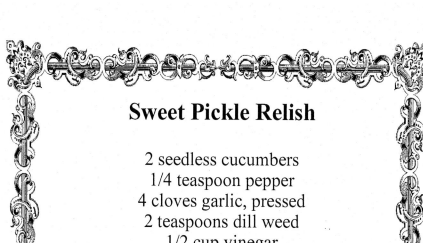

Sweet Pickle Relish

2 seedless cucumbers
1/4 teaspoon pepper
4 cloves garlic, pressed
2 teaspoons dill weed
1/2 cup vinegar
1 cup water
1 teaspoon lemon juice
1 teaspoon salt
4 Tablespoons sugar

Peel cucumbers. Finely chop and combine in medium saucepan with remaining ingredients. Cook over medium heat, stirring occasionally, until water is reduced.

Chill before serving.

Honey Butter

1/2 cup butter
1/2 cup canola oil
1/2 cup honey

Combine in blender. Blend for 30 seconds. Transfer to airtight container and refrigerate.

Mayonnaise

1-1/4 cups canola oil
2 egg whites
1 teaspoon ground mustard
1/2 teaspoon salt
3/4 teaspoon Tabasco
1 teaspoon sugar
3 Tablespoons lemon juice

Place 1/4 cup of oil in a blender, together with egg whites, mustard, salt, Tabasco and sugar.

Blend ingredients until thoroughly combined. While blender is still running, gradually add 1/2 cup of oil, then lemon juice, then remaining oil.

Blend until thickened. Keep refrigerated in an air-tight container.

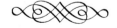

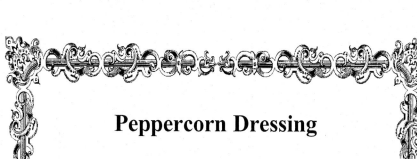

Peppercorn Dressing

1 cup plain, nonfat yogurt (no xanthan gum)
1/4 cup vinegar
1-1/2 teaspoons lemon juice
1/3 cup parmesan
1/2 teaspoon coarsely grated peppercorns
1/2 teaspoon garlic powder

Combine ingredients in mason jar. Cover and shake until thoroughly combined. Serve over salad or vegetables.

Parmesan Dressing

1-1/2 cups yogurt, drained
1/3 cup sugar
2 Tablespoons vinegar
1/2 cup parmesan cheese
1/4 teaspoon salt (optional)
1/4 cup finely chopped onion

Combine ingredients in a blender. Mix well and use over salad or vegetables.

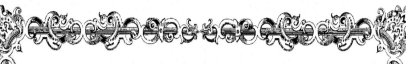

Dijon Dressing

2 Tablespoons vinegar
4 Tablespoons oil
3 Tablespoons coarse Dijon mustard
1/4 cup onion, finely chopped
2 cloves garlic, pressed
1/8 teaspoon pepper

Combine in a small mixing bowl. Stir until ingredients are well combined. Let stand 10-15 minutes to allow the ingredients to blend. Stir again before serving.

Lemon Dressing

2 Tablespoons lemon juice
2 Tablespoons canola oil
1/2 teaspoon garlic powder
1/2 teaspoon onion
1/8 teaspoon salt
1/8 teaspoon pepper

Combine ingredients in a small mixing bowl. Blend well and toss into salad.

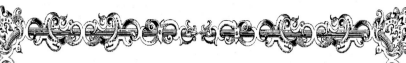

Honey Mustard Dressing

2 Tablespoons smooth Dijon mustard
2 Tablespoons vinegar
4 Tablespoons canola oil
2 teaspoons honey
1/4 teaspoon garlic powder
1/8 teaspoon pepper

Combine ingredients in a small mixing bowl. Blend with a fork, then let stand 15 minutes to allow the mustard to absorb the ingredients and flavors. Blend again with fork and toss into salad.

Italian Dressing

1/4 cup vinegar
1/2 cup oil
1/2 teaspoon garlic powder
1/2 teaspoon onion powder
1/8 teaspoon pepper
1/2 teaspoon dried oregano

Combine ingredients in mason jar or cruet. Cover and shake until blended. Toss into salad.

Caesar Italian Dressing

Italian Dressing (see previous recipe)
1/4 cup parmesan cheese

Combine ingredients in mason jar or cruet.
Cover and shake until blended. Let stand
10 minutes. This will give the flavors a
chance to blend with the cheese. Shake
again. Toss into salad.

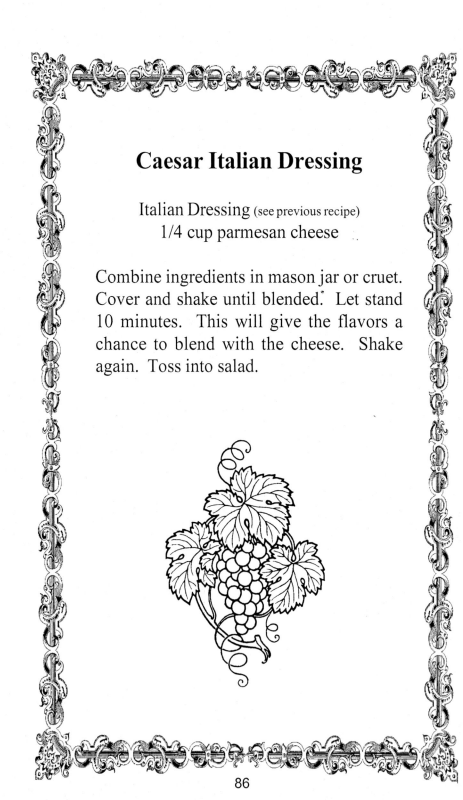

Desserts

Frozen Cherry Yogurt

1 1/4 cup cherry juice
2 teaspoons lemon juice
1/2 cup sugar
1 cup plain, nonfat yogurt (no xanthan gum)

Combine juices and sugar in a medium mixing bowl. Blend with whisk until sugar is dissolved.

Add yogurt and continue to stir until ingredients are fully blended. Transfer to ice cream maker, freezing for about 35 minutes or until desired consistency is reached.

Serve immediately or store frozen in an airtight container.

Makes about 3 cups.

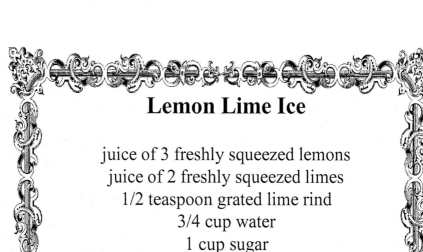

Lemon Lime Ice

juice of 3 freshly squeezed lemons
juice of 2 freshly squeezed limes
1/2 teaspoon grated lime rind
3/4 cup water
1 cup sugar

Juice should come to about 3/4 cup total. Combine all ingredients in a mixing bowl. Stir until sugar is dissolved, about one minute.

Transfer to an ice cream maker, freezing for about 25 minutes or until desired consistency is reached. Serve immediately. Makes about 3 cups.

Wild Cherry Ice

1-1/2 cups cherry juice
1/2 cup water
4 teaspoons lemon juice
1/4 cup sugar

Combine ingredients in medium mixing bowl. Stir until sugar is dissolved, about 1 minute. Transfer to ice cream maker, freezing for about 20 minutes or until desired consistency is reached. Blend with whisk. and serve immediately.

Strawberry Fluff

2 egg whites
3/4 cup powdered sugar
1 pound strawberries
1-1/2 Tablespoons lemon juice
2 strawberries for garnish

Remove tops from strawberries. Set aside.

In a medium mixing bowl, beat egg whites with an electric mixer until stiff, about 2 minutes. Continue beating, gradually adding sugar, until smooth.

Place in a blender. Add strawberries and lemon juice. Pulse blend until smooth. Pour into dessert dishes and chill for 1-1/2 hours.

Serve garnished with fresh strawberry slices. This tasty dessert has a delicate, creamy consistency.

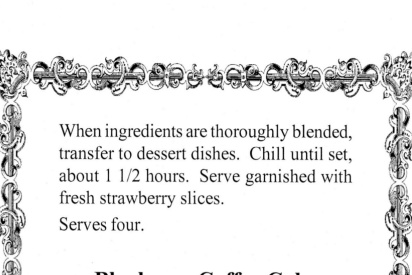

When ingredients are thoroughly blended, transfer to dessert dishes. Chill until set, about 1 1/2 hours. Serve garnished with fresh strawberry slices.

Serves four.

Blueberry Coffee Cake

2 egg whites
1/3 cup sugar
1/2 teaspoon baking powder
3/4 cup flour
1/4 cup margarine, softened
1 teaspoon lemon juice
1 teaspoon vanilla extract
1 cup blueberries

Preheat oven to 350 degrees. Lightly coat a 9 x 5 x 3 bread pan with canola oil; set aside.

In a medium mixing bowl, beat the egg whites with an electric mixer until peaks form. Add sugar gradually, continuing to beat with mixer. Egg whites will become stiff and shiny.

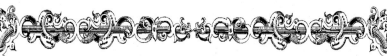

Continue beating with mixer, gradually adding baking powder, flour, margarine, lemon juice and vanilla extract, until these ingredients are thoroughly combined.

Fold in blueberries. Transfer to bread pan. Bake 20 minutes or until the sides brown and a toothpick inserted in the center comes out clean.

Cool and cut into squares. Serves four.

Ginger Coffee Cake

2 cups flour
1/2 cup brown sugar
2 teaspoons baking powder
1/2 teaspoon salt
1 cup skim milk
2 egg whites
3/4 cup dates or prunes, chopped
2 Tablespoons margarine, softened
2 Tablespoons ginger, freshly grated

Preheat oven to 350 degrees. Lightly coat a 9-inch round cake pan with canola oil; set aside.

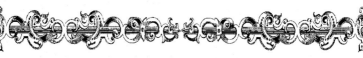

In a large mixing bowl, combine flour, brown sugar, baking powder, and salt.

While blending with electric mixer, add milk, egg whites, prunes, margarine and ginger. Blend until ingredients are well combined and batter is formed. Transfer to cake pan.

Bake for 30-35 minutes or until surface is golden brown and toothpick inserted in center comes out clean. Cool before serving. Serves six.

Basic Vanilla Pudding

3 Tablespoons cornstarch
1/2 cup sugar
1 cup skim milk
3 egg whites
1 teaspoon vanilla extract

Blend all ingredients with a whisk until smooth. Cook in a non-stick saucepan over medium to high heat, stirring frequently, until mixture begins to thicken, about 20 minutes.

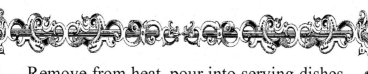

Remove from heat, pour into serving dishes and allow to cool. Pudding will thicken more as it cools. Serve warm or chilled.

Pearboat Salad

2 ripe pears
2 teaspoons orange juice
4 oz. low-fat cream cheese (no xanthan gum)
1/3 cup dried cherries, chopped
1 Tablespoon cherry juice
4 dried cherries (for garnish)

Halve and core pears. Hollow to 1/2" thickness, setting aside removed pulp. Place pear halves in a locking zipper bag with orange juice. Shake until fully coated. This will help keep the pears from turning brown. Remove pear halves from bag and set aside.

Pour remaining orange juice from bag into a mixing bowl. Chop the removed pear pulp and add to the mixing bowl. Add the cream cheese, chopped dried cherries and cherry juice. Stir with a large spoon until blended.

Spoon into pear halves and top each with a dried cherry.
Serves four.

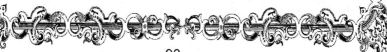

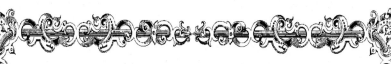

Blackberry Yogurt

1 cup fresh blackberries
2 Tablespoons sugar
1 Tablespoon water
2 cups plain, nonfat yogurt (no xanthan gum)

Combine blackberries, sugar and water in a mixing bowl. Stir until sugar is dissolved, lightly mashing berries. Fold into yogurt and serve garnished with fresh berries. Serves two.

Variation: Replace blackberries with raspberries or a mixture of both.

Peach Yogurt

1 peach
1 Tablespoon sugar
1/2 teaspoon lemon juice
1 cup plain, nonfat yogurt (no xanthan gum)

Peel peach. Remove pit and chop. Place in saucepan with sugar and lemon juice. Cook over medium heat, stirring well, until sugar dissolves and liquid thickens to a syrup. Remove from heat. Chill. Gently fold into yogurt.

Serves two.

Strawberry Yogurt

1/2 pint strawberries
2 Tablespoons sugar
1-1/2 cups plain, nonfat yogurt
(no xanthan gum)

Cut tops from strawberries and discard. Cut strawberries into small pieces (quarters or eighths). Place in mixing bowl. Add sugar.

Fold 2-3 minutes until sugar is dissolved and syrup forms. Adding liquid is not necessary.

Fold into yogurt.

Serves two.

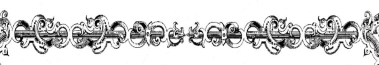

Cranberry Yogurt

1 cup fresh cranberries
1 cup water
1/3 cup sugar
1-1/2 cups plain, nonfat yogurt
(no xanthan gum)

Combine cranberries, water and sugar in a small saucepan. Bring to a boil, then reduce heat. Simmer, stirring occasionally, for 15 minutes or until thickened.

Remove from heat, cool and chill. Fold into yogurt. Serves two.

Cherry Pudding Crisp

1 cup crushed corn flakes
1/2 cup brown sugar
1/3 cup margarine, melted
3 Tablespoons cornstarch
1/2 cup sugar
1 cup skim milk
3 egg whites
1 teaspoon vanilla extract
1 cup pitted cherries

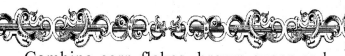

Combine corn flakes, brown sugar and margarine, stirring with a fork until flakesare evenly coated. Place in bottom of four dessert dishes and set aside.

Combine cornstarch, sugar milk, egg whites and vanilla. Blend with a whisk until smooth. Cook in a saucepan over medium heat, until it begins to thicken. Stir in cherries, continuing to stir. Re-heat to the boiling point.

Remove from heat, pour into dessert dishes over corn flake mixture. Allow to cool. Pudding will thicken as it cools. Serve warm or chilled.

Rice Pudding Fluff

3/4 cups chopped walnuts
1-1/2 cups cooked rice
3/4 cup raisins or chopped prunes
1/2 cup brown sugar, packed
2 egg whites

Preheat oven to 350 degrees. Lightly coat a 9 x 5 x 3 bread pan with canola oil. Set aside.

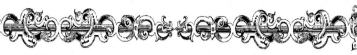

Combine all ingredients in a mixing bowl, stirring with a spoon until evenly distributed. The brown sugar and egg whiteswill make a sort of syrup.

Pack firmly in bread pan. Bake for 40 minutes. Remove from oven. Cool 10 minutes, fluff with fork and serve.

Pierogies

2 cups flour
1/2 teaspoon salt
1 egg
4 egg whites
1 teaspoon water
3 peaches
1 Tablespoon sugar
1/2 teaspoon lemon juice
1/2 cup plain, nonfat yogurt (no xanthan gum)

Combine flour, salt and eggs. Mix by hand, adding the teaspoon of water to any remaining dry spots. Knead with floured hands about two minutes or until the dough begins to lose its sticky feel. Refrigerate for 1/2 hour.

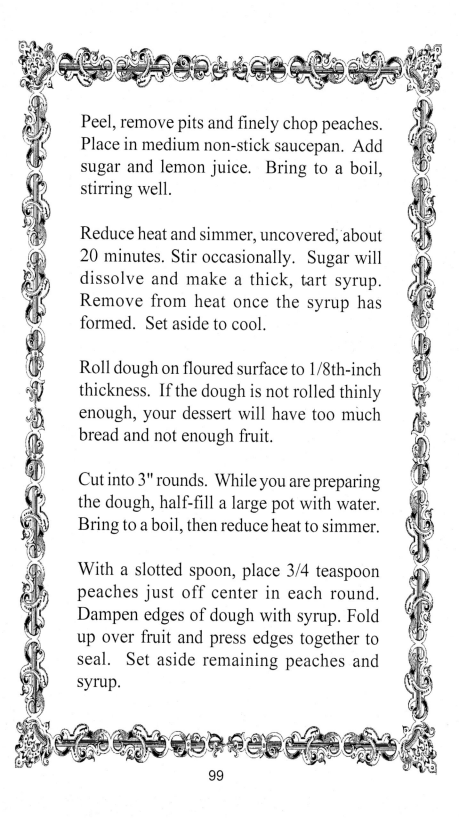

Peel, remove pits and finely chop peaches. Place in medium non-stick saucepan. Add sugar and lemon juice. Bring to a boil, stirring well.

Reduce heat and simmer, uncovered, about 20 minutes. Stir occasionally. Sugar will dissolve and make a thick, tart syrup. Remove from heat once the syrup has formed. Set aside to cool.

Roll dough on floured surface to 1/8th-inch thickness. If the dough is not rolled thinly enough, your dessert will have too much bread and not enough fruit.

Cut into 3" rounds. While you are preparing the dough, half-fill a large pot with water. Bring to a boil, then reduce heat to simmer.

With a slotted spoon, place 3/4 teaspoon peaches just off center in each round. Dampen edges of dough with syrup. Fold up over fruit and press edges together to seal. Set aside remaining peaches and syrup.

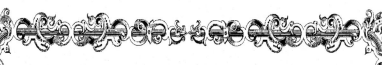

Drop pierogies into gently boiling water. Cook about 15 minutes, until they rise to the surface. Remove with slotted spoon and gently place in colander to drain. Set aside to cool.

Mix remaining peaches and syrup with yogurt. Fold yogurt mixture into pierogies until lightly coated. Serve.
Makes 2 dozen.

Baked Apples

3 small apples, peeled, cored and finely chopped
1 cup cooked white rice
1/2 cup brown sugar, packed
2 egg whites
1/2 cup white rice flour
1 teaspoon baking powder
3 teaspoons lemon juice
1/4 teaspoon nutmeg
1/4 teaspoon cinnamon

Preheat oven to 375 degrees. Lightly coat a small casserole dish with canola oil. Set aside.

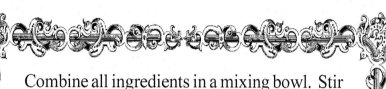

Combine all ingredients in a mixing bowl. Stir until thoroughly combined. Place in casserole dish and bake 30 minutes or until surface has a crusty texture. Remove from oven, cool for about 15 minutes, stir and serve. Makes four servings.

Almond Crisps

1/2 cup margarine
1 cup sugar
2 egg whites
1-1/2 cup white rice flour
1 teaspoon baking powder
1 teaspoon almond extract
2/3 cup finely chopped almonds

Preheat oven to 375 degrees. Lightly coat a cookie sheet with canola oil. Set aside.

Combine all ingredients in mixing bowl. Blend with a hand mixer on high about 3 minutes or until texture is thick and fluffy. Spoon by teaspoonsful onto cookie sheet.

Bake 15 minutes or until edges are browned. Remove from oven and cool completely before removing from cookie sheet. This will help to prevent breakage. Makes about 3 dozen.

Metric
Conversions

1 pound	.4536 kg
1 ounce (weight)	28.35 grams
1 cup	.2365 liter
2 cups (1 pint)	.473 liter
4 cups (1 quart)	.946 liter
4 quarts (1 gallon)	3.784 liters
1 teaspoon	5 ml
1 Tablespoon	15 ml
1 fluid ounce (1/8 cup)	30 ml

Fahrenheit is converted to degrees Celsius as follows:
1. Begin with degrees Fahrenheit
2. Subtract 32
3. Multiply by 5
4. Divide by 9

Salicylates
Following is a list of some medications which contain salicylates:

Aspirin
Anacin
Anaflex
Arthritis Pain Formula
Anthropan
Aspergum
Bayer Aspirin
Bufferin
Cope
Doan's Regular Strength Tablets
Ecotrin
Empirin
Gensan
Healthprin
Mono-Gesic
Tricosal
Trilisate

• A more comprehensive list may be obtained from your doctor or local pharmacist.

Legumes
(Relatively High in Purines and Not Allowed)

adzuki beans
black beans
black-eyed peas (cowpeas, black-eyed beans)
butter beans
cannellini
chick-peas
cranberry beans (not to be confused with cranberries)
fava beans (broad beans)
flageolets
garbanzo beans
great northern beans
kidney beans
lentils
lima beans
mung beans
navy beans
peanuts
peas
pinto beans
red beans
soy beans
split peas
white beans

Bibliography

The information contained in this book was obtained from the following sources:

Aesoph, Lauri M., *How to Eat Away Arthritis*, Revised and Expanded, 1996 Prentice Hall

Arthritis Foundation, "Gout" brochure, 1999, Arthritis Foundation

Arthritis Foundation, "Diet and your Arthritis," brochure, 1999, Arthritis Foundation

Basic Facts About Processed Free Glutamic Acid (MSG), Truth in Labeling Campaign website: www.truthinlabeling.org

Chang, David J., "Of all the ginned joints....," *Patient Care*, March 15, 1996, v.30, n. 5, p. 182 (3)

Ellman, Michael, H. M.D., "Treating acute gouty arthritis," *The Journal of Musculoskeletal Medicine*, March 1992, pp. 71-74

Emmerson, Bryan T. M.D., Ph. D., "The Management of Gout," *The New England Journal of Medicine*, Volume 334 Number 7, February 1996, pp 445-451

Flieger, Ken, "Getting to know Gout," *FDA Consumer*, March 1995 v29 n2

Forbes Digital Tool: "Cool-Lay off the sheep heart and smelt, or else!," wysiwyg://53/http://www.forbes.com/tool/html/97/sep/0920/side2.htm, June 21, 2000, Forbes.com

Gold, Mark, "Monosodium Glutamate, " 5/8/95 website*: http://www.holisticmed.com/msg/msg-mark.txt   *Article also contains extensive list of sources for more reading on the subject of MSG

Gott, Peter, "Gout may be related to medicines," *The Dominion Post*, April 27, 2001

Harness, R. Angus; Elion, Gertrude B.; Zoellner, Nepomuk, *Purine and Pyrimidine Metabolism in Man VII, Part A: Chemotherapy, ATP Depletion and Gout*, 1991, Plenum Press, pp. 3, 139-142, 181, 185-203, 217-221, 227-230, 341-344

Lipetz, Philip, M.D., *The Good Calorie Diet*, 1994, HarperCollins Publishers, pp 188-189

Margen, Sheldon, M.D., *The Wellness Encyclopedia of Food and Nutrition*, 1992, University of CA at Berkeley, Health Letter Associates, pp. 91-94, 348-358

Martinez-Maldonado, Manuel, "How to avoid Kidney Stones, *Saturday Evenilng Post*, Sept.-Oct. 1995, v.267, n. 5, p. 36(3)

MotherNature.com Health Encyclopedia, Low-Purine Diet, http://www.mothernature.com/ency/Diet/Low-Purine_Diet.asp, 1998, HealthNotes, Inc.

National Institute of Arthritis and Musculoskeletal Skin Diseases, "Questions and Answers About Gout," fact sheet

Pennington, Jean A.T., *Bowes & Church's Food Values of Portions Commonly Used*, Edition 17, 1998 Lippincott-Raven, p.391

Porter, Roy and Rousseau, G.S., *Gout, the Patrician Malady*, 1998 Yale University Press

Pritikin, Nathan, *The Pritikin Promise*, 1983, Simon and Schuster, pp. 110-111

Purine Research Society, Bethesda, MD, Web-site: http://www2.dgsys.com/~purine/

"Salicylates-oral," Health Central- General Encycopedia website: http://www.webrx.com

Sauber, Colleen M., "Still painful after all these years. (gout)," *Harvard Health Letter*, June 1995, v20, n8, p. 6 (3).

Saunders, Carol S., "Gout: Applying Current Knowledge," *Patient Care*, May 30, 1998, v32 n10 p 125

Souci, S.W.; Fachmann, H.; Kraut; *Food Composition and Nutrition Tables*, CRC Press, Medpharm, Scientific Publishers Stuttgart 2000, 6th Revised and Complete Edition

Steyer, Robert, "Arthritis Sufferers put up a spirited fight against chronic pain," *St. Louis Post-Dispatch*, Feb. 14, 1999

Strange, Carolyn J., "Coping with Arthritis in its many forms, *FDA Consumer*, March 1996, pp. 17-21

Talboth, John H; Yu, Ts'al-Fan, M.D., *Gout and Uric Acid Metabolism*, 1976, Stratton Intercontinental Medical Book Corp.

Wolfram, G. and Colling, M., *Z. Ernahrungswiss*, 1987, vol. 26, pp 205-13

Lab testing for purine levels in the following foods was provided by Biogen Laboratory Developments, LLC in Gresham, Oregon:

Jicama
Okra
Beets
Grits
Broccoli
Corn Flakes
Turnips
Water Chestnuts
Collard Greens

All items were found to be low in purines at less than 50 mg per 100 g, except broccoli, which was reported at about 71 mg per 100 g.

Purine values tested were "reported as uric acid derived from total converted purine +/- 20 mg." Broccoli was tested both raw and cooked; grits were tested after preparation according to package instructions.

INDEX

INDEX

INDEX

Information Resources

To find out more about gout, sources of information include:

Arthritis Foundation
1330 West Peachtree Street
Atlanta, GA
U.S.A.
(404) 872-7100
(800) 283-7800

National Institute of Arthritis and Musculoskeletal and Skin
Diseases (NIAMS) Information Clearinghouse
1 AMS Circle
Bethesda, MD   20892-3675
U.S.A.
Phone: (301) 495-4484 or (877) 22-NIAMS (toll free)
TTY: (301) 565-2966
Fax: (301) 718-6366

Purine Research Society
5424 Beech Ave.
Bethesda, MD 20814-1730
U.S.A.
E-mail: purine@erols.com
Web-site: http://www2.dgsys.com/~purine/

About the Author

Jodi Schneiter holds a Bachelors degree in Social Sciences and history, as well as an Associates degree in Liberal Arts. A member of Phi Theta Kappa, the national honor society for two year colleges, she has been named in two annual editions of the *National Dean's List*.

Also by Jodi Schneiter:

Gout Hater's Cookbook:
Recipes Lower in Purines and Lower in Fat
Modified Purine Diet recipes, Lower in Purines and Lower in Fat;
Features Lists of Foods Lowest,
Relatively High and Highest in Purines

Gout Hater's Cookbook III:
The Low Purine Diet Cookbook
Restricted Purine Diet, Complies with
Modified and Restricted Purine Diets
Features Lists of Foods Allowed and Not Allowed;
Showing Lowest, Relatively High and Highest in Purines;
Features Suggestions for Holiday Dishes